7
Health Tips
for a
Fast Paced
Society

Ana Gonzalez

Mill City Press, Inc.
322 First Avenue N, 5th floor
Minneapolis, MN 55401
612.455.2293
www.millcitypublishing.com

The content of this book is for general instruction only. Each person's physical, emotional, and spiritual condition is unique. The instruction in this book is not intended to replace or interrupt the reader's relationship with a physician or other professional. Please consult your doctor for matters pertaining to your specific health and diet.

ISBN-13: 978-1-63413-481-1
LCCN: 2015905332

Printed in the United States of America

I dedicate this book with love and gratitude to my beloved husband John who has been with me during all the ups and downs of life with so much courage, strength and faith.

Ana Gonzalez

CONTENTS

ACKNOWLEDGMENTS

I would like to thank very specially Joshua Rosenthal, founder, director and primary teacher of the Institute for Integrative Nutrition in New York. Not only has he inspired me to write this book but he has been an outstanding teacher and compassionate listener.

I also thank Lindsey Smith for guiding me through, every step of the way.

I am most grateful to my nephew and niece, Silvio and Sonia Cruz very specially for their invaluable help and input in making this book come alive with the photography, editing and graphic design.

Thank you, Creator of our Universe for having guided me in this direction.

INTRODUCTION

At the age of 27, I decided to come to America from Spain because I felt I needed a new beginning, whereupon I embarked on my new adventure.

I had to adapt to my new home and I encountered many wonderful people along this path.

I met my husband John when I was 29 and at age 30 we were happily married and all was well.

Four years later, there was suddenly an abrupt change in our harmony and well being. We were about to take a flight to our vacation destination and I fell ill and was hospitalized. The diagnosis was a brain hemorrhage which lead to a stroke.

After this event and upon my recovery and treatment, I had to rethink everything that I thought I knew. I started to observe that most of the lovely people around me were as caught up in the race of modern society as I was. One thing I noticed in retrospect was that history has a way of repeating itself.

My thought is simple now. Life is a gift to us and as recipients of such, we must learn to listen to our bodies and take care of them.

The healing ideas I give the readers in this book have been based on my own experience towards health. They are listed in order of my view of importance. First, we breathe, then we drink and if all the steps are done correctly, a smile will surely follow.

Although our society is geared to move very fast indeed, my hope is that these 7 very simple tips help everyone to stay healthy and happy through this amazing journey we call "life".

Chapter One
BREATHE

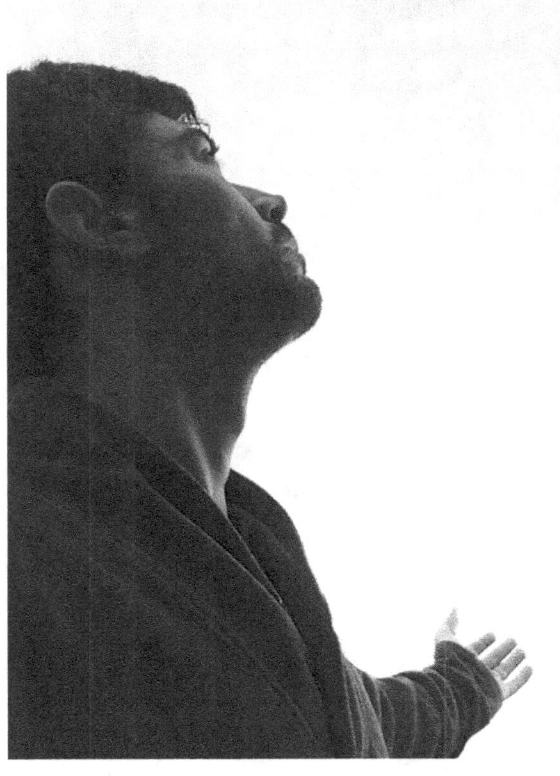

We have read in many books that the body is the temple of the soul. Look at all the religious churches and temples in the world. They are so beautiful, artistic, clean and spiritual. If we humans are capable of taking such good care of those temples, we should also be able to do the same with our body temples, shouldn't we?

Breathing is the first and most important thing we do to stay alive. We can be without drinking for some time and without eating for even longer periods of time, but breathing needs to be done constantly,

Normally, in our society, when we wake up in the morning, we run to the shower, brush our teeth, get dressed and head out to work. We do not pay attention to the way we're breathing during that time.

If we stop for a minute and pay attention to our breath, we can feel that it may be rather shallow, coming in and out of our nose with no full, deep breaths. This shallow breathing is not enough to nourish all the cells in our bodies, so we become stressed right away while we commute to work. We get aggravated when bumping into other people in the subways when the cars are too full, when the trains are delayed because of signal problems, when we are caught in traffic jams and trying to get to work on time, etc.

However, if upon awakening, we focus on our breathing while doing our routines, things will start improving. If we start by breathing deeply, in through our nose and into our lungs and further down into our abdomen and expanding it, and then, breathing out slowly, contracting our abdomen and expelling the air through our lungs and then through our nose or mouth, our cells will be nourished.

I recommend starting slowly and being mindful of your breathing. As you increase your breathing awareness and extend the time of slow, deep breathing, you will feel a subtle difference by being more centered and your mind will be more peaceful. You will start to see things in a lighter and brighter way, feel more positive and then, somehow, the day will feel smoother and your stress level will decline.

I leave the counting of the breath to what is comfortable for each individual. To me, inhaling deeply to a count of five, filling my belly like a balloon and then exhaling deeply to a count of five is a comfortable choice. Some people choose other ways of deep breathing, for example, to inhale to a count of four, hold the breath to a count of seven and exhale to a count of eight. This method is believed to improve digestion and circulation.

You can also visualize something beautiful while doing this exercise like breathing in golden light and breathing out any aches, pains and negative thoughts.
Your body and mind will tell you what feels good. Let's practice our breathing.

Chapter Two
DRINK

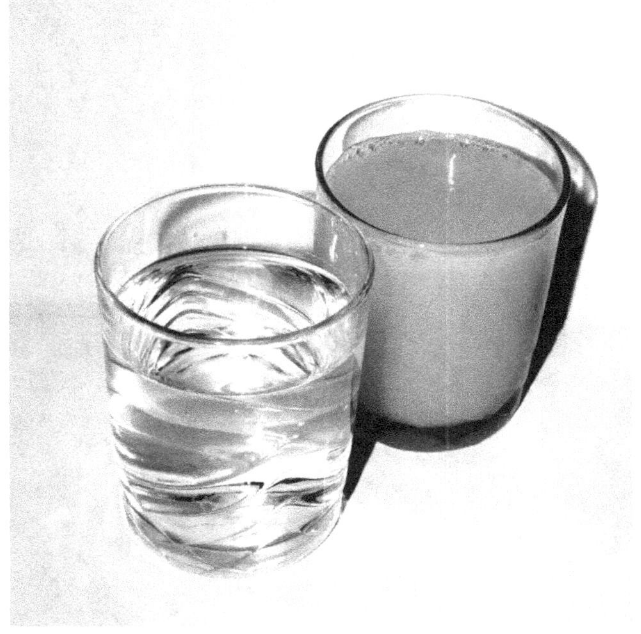

The second most important thing we have to do is to drink.

Water is the best choice. Water hydrates us, cleanses our bodies and keeps all our cells alive since our bodies are about 90% water when we are born and 70% as adults.

When we do not drink enough water, we do not eliminate toxins well, our skin ages quickly, our bones start to feel painful, our minds are burdened with negative thoughts and we do not feel flexible, we feel stiff.

Water is truly a miracle in our lives. We should honor it, respect it, preserve it and drink it with gratitude.

Have you ever thought about how humble water is? It can have the strength to destroy us with its awesome power and yet it will do the humblest of things such as eliminating our waste down a toilet, leaving everything clean behind it.

Nowadays, some sources of our drinking water are polluted so it is important to have good water filtration systems at home or to buy bottled water, preferably in glass bottles because some plastic bottles can leach chemicals into the water even if the source is clean.

Normally, eight glasses of water are recommended throughout the day. Sometimes, there is no time to drink so much and some people feel comfortable with four or five cups instead. A good idea is to keep water next to your work post and sip some as needed.

We may also drink herbal teas and unsweetened juices. The less sugar we consume, the better we'll feel so it's important to read labels. Coconut water is a good source of hydration and it replenishes our electrolytes. Although it has some natural sugar, it is less sweet than soft drinks and sweetened beverages and is definitely my best choice after water to stay hydrated.

My favorite herbal teas are rooibos tea for its great antioxidant capacity, green tea for its compounds known as polyphenols and antioxidants known to lower cancer and cardiovascular disease. However, although green tea has many health properties, some people feel nauseous if they drink it on an empty stomach in the morning. I'm one of those people, so it may be best to drink it after or during a meal. Chamomile tea with anise is another of my favorites because it calms the mind and helps with digestion. Mint tea is also good for aiding in digestion.

Many of us like to have some sort of milk in the morning with our breakfast and added to our tea or coffee. Although some people enjoy cow's milk, today there is a tendency towards almond, soy or rice milk instead. Also hemp and coconut milk are on the rise. Goat's milk is used less, probably because of its strong taste. My husband and I personally prefer unsweetened rice and quinoa milk. We have noticed that cow's milk affects our breathing and almond and soy milks do not agree with our bodies so much either. We are all different so what's good for me may not be good for you. The best is to experiment and see what type of milk is better for you.

Coffee is many people's first choice for breakfast and throughout the day. A cup or two may be beneficial due to its antioxidant properties but if you drink a lot of coffee, it will dehydrate your body, so make sure to increase your water intake if you absolutely must drink more than two cups a day.

Sometimes, we have social drinking which often involves alcoholic beverages. Red wine is probably the best choice because it contains resveratrol which is good for the heart. An occasional glass is alright for whoever can tolerate it but not too much of it is good because all alcohol converts to sugar which can be detrimental to our overall health.

Beer also has its mild benefits if not abused. Some people believe it may aid our kidneys from developing kidney stones. Others are saying that it improves our memory.

As far as spirit drinks go, my parents occasionally had a little shot of whisky on Sundays after lunch because they believed it was good for the heart. Everything in moderation though when it comes to drinking alcoholic beverages, that is, the less, the better.

Chapter Three
EAT

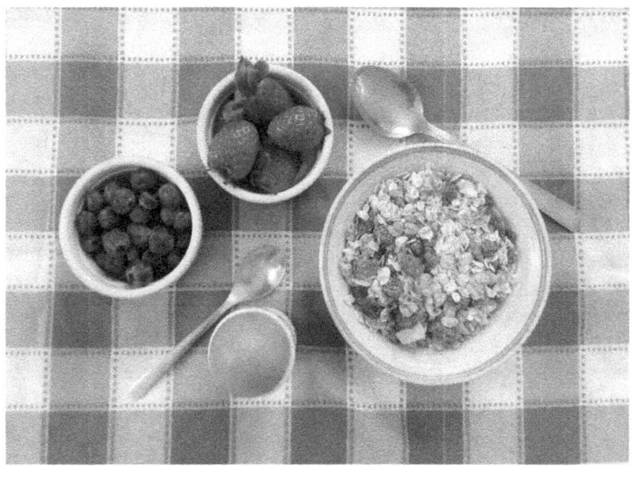

Eating is the third most important thing we must do so we should try to eat as much healthy food as possible.

I feel that the most important foods to eat are vegetables, especially the dark and leafy ones like kale, collard greens, bok choy and broccoli rabe. Broccoli is another favorite veggie. These foods are packed with vitamins and minerals and they help prevent cancer, cleanse our bodies and build our immune systems.
Although spinach and swiss chard are also very healthy for us, we should consume them in moderation due to their oxalic acid content which could lead to kidney stone formation in some people and depletion of calcium from our bones.

We should enjoy a nice salad every day, especially with romaine lettuce which is healthy for the heart and we can add a lovely cucumber which helps us stay hydrated. Some celery may help lower high blood pressure, and a few olives will keep inflammation down. Then, a splash of extra virgin olive oil will give us antioxidant protection. Not bad for a salad !

Other colored vegetables are also very healthy for us such as root vegetables like carrots, turnips and beets, packed with vitamins and minerals.

The allium family: onions, garlic, scallions and leeks are great for the heart, help lower cholesterol, are good for the immune system and protect us from cancer, so if you can, add them to your cooking as much as possible. Your food will taste very flavorful.

We should not forget our lovely orange vegetables: pumpkins, butternut squash, spaghetti squash and acorn squash, all filled with beta carotene. Yams are fine to have once in a while. These foods are a favorite during the colder months.

The nightshade family is also needed, but in less quantities for some of us who notice a little pain in our bones if we consume them in excess. Arthritis sufferers beware of them because they may cause inflammation in your body. Your condition will be aggravated by them. They include potatoes, tomatoes, eggplants and peppers (green, yellow, orange and red). For those who tolerate them well, they have phytochemicals that protect your cells from damage and tomatoes are rich in the carotenoid lycopene.

My quickest cooking method is to steam, saute or boil my vegetables and then dress them with extra virgin olive oil, a simple solution for a busy schedule.

I believe the veggies may be accompanied by healthy grains such as brown rice, quinoa or soba noodles. You can make large quantities to last for a few days in the refrigerator. I simply boil them.

You may also make healthy legumes to accompany your veggies. My choices are black beans, aduki beans and lentils. Other people prefer other legumes which agree more with their digestive systems, such as white or navy beans and chickpeas.

We may also add to our dishes the healing and immune protecting mushrooms, especially maitake, reishi and shiitake.

Let's add some animal protein if we are not totally vegetarian. How about some nice wild caught salmon or sardines, packed with omega 3 fatty acids and less mercury than other larger fish? By the way, the benefits of Omega 3s are keeping the heart, the eyes and the brain healthy. These fish are anti-inflammatory. I stir fry mine with olive oil and a little water. Delicious!

A piece of organic, grass fed beef no bigger than the size of the palm of your hand will give you protein, iron, zinc and vitamin B12. Poultry meat such as chicken breast or turkey which has tryptophan, an amino acid that our bodies use to make serotonin, a neurotransmitter that makes us feel good, are great alternatives if you do not tolerate red meat well.

We need our healthy fats too: raw nuts such as walnuts, pumpkin seeds, cashews, almonds, avocados and oil especially olive and coconut oils, in moderate quantities.

Whole, organic eggs are also good for us, if we can tolerate them well, because they are a wonderful source of protein and contain the nine essential amino acids. The yolk of the egg is especially beneficial for our eyes, heart, nervous system and brain.

It is also necessary to have fruit, but at separate intervals from our main meals because they can interfere with our digestion.
Apples are a winner as well as all the berry family, which are less sweet than other fruits and can be well tolerated by people with diabetes. Grapefruits are also less sweet but people who take certain medications cannot eat them because they interfere with the absorption of the medication.

In the spring and summer months, we may enjoy our papayas, bananas and the melon family which all help cool our bodies. Watermelon has plenty of lycopene, a powerful antioxidant which may protect us from prostate, stomach and lung cancers. Pineapples, kiwis and guavas are great because they have vitamin C and pineapples have bromelain which is an anti inflammatory enzyme that aids digestion. Cherries are in season and are very good to counteract gout.

In the fall and winter, we like our pomegranates, plums, oranges and clementines to increase our vitamin C which help our immune systems stay strong. Pears are great for their high content in fiber.

You may have noticed that in my recommendations I have not mentioned refined carbohydrates such as white rice or pasta or even bread and the reason is that these foods convert to sugar quickly in our bodies and they lack the nutrients of whole grains. Also, most breads have gluten and nowadays there is a larger group of people becoming intolerant to gluten.

Milk derived foods such as cheese or yoghurt may be eaten in moderation. In both cases, it is preferable to eat goat or sheep products because they are easier to digest and are more similar to human milk than cow's milk.

Sea vegetables should be an important addition to our diet. Dulse, kelp, hijiki, nori, arame and kombu protect us from radiation and environmental pollution. I add plenty of dulse and kelp to my cooking.

Remember to add your herbs and spices to condiment your food. A very healthy and cleansing variety are: fennel, parsley, cumin, ginger, coriander, turmeric, thyme, rosemary, oregano, cayenne pepper, cinnamon and bay leaves.

Breakfasts should be hearty. Eggs and fish may be eaten some days and oats with milk and fruit may be eaten on other days. Some people enjoy plain yoghurt with berries and granola. We should add plenty of flax meal to our breakfast because it helps with bowel movements and is packed with omega 3 fatty acids.

Lunches should be hearty too. In the winter months, a lovely bean or chicken soup will warm our bodies and as a second dish, we may eat our choice of vegetables, grains and/or animal or plant proteins.

Dinners should be small. At night, it is healthier to eat little food so that we can have a restful sleep and feel more energized when waking up in the morning. .

Also, of you can, try to buy organic and locally grown food as much as possible. They do not contain harmful pesticides and the beef, white meat and eggs do not contain hormones which may also be harmful to us. Local food does not need as much refrigeration time and is therefore fresher.

To end this chapter, I recommend that preferably, you purchase cooking pots and pans that are made of glass or stainless steel instead of those made of aluminum or Teflon. I believe that aluminum and Teflon materials are questionable to our health because they may leach into our food during the cooking process.

Experiment and see what feels best for you!

Chapter Four
EXERCISE

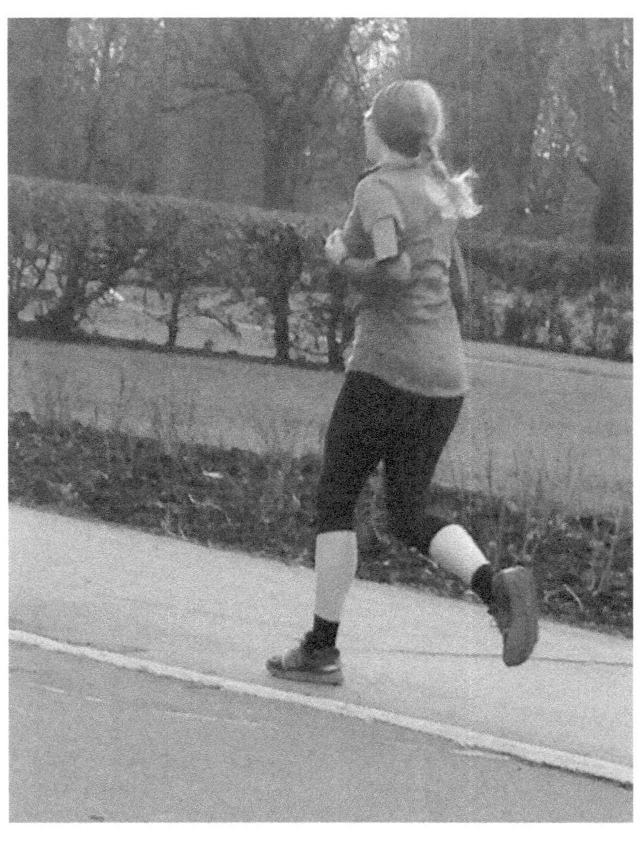

In order for our bodies to stay supple, agile and young, it is important to exercise every day.

If we commute by subway, it is good to walk up stairs or escalators to get our hearts moving. For those who drive, it is good to park your car a few blocks from your job and then walk there. At lunch break, it is important to walk at least about 30 minutes briskly if possible but try not to breathe too deeply if you're in an area that has pollution or smog. The best choice would be to walk in a park, but not everyone has that luxury to be close to one.

Also, at work, if sitting for long periods of time, it is prudent to stand up every hour and walk around the office and then go back to work. We are not meant to sit all day. Standing is healthier for us.

After work, many people like to go to the gym and work out. That is a wonderful choice. Others prefer to do yoga or pilates to stretch and relax their minds and bodies. Others prefer martial arts to keep them strong, focused and motivated. I like to do Tai Chi and Qi Gong practice. It balances my body, mind and spirit and the movements strengthen my inner core and take away any aches and pains I may have at the moment. For me and many other people, this is a very complete way to stay healthy.

Swimming is a fabulous way to move our bodies and to keep them strong and supple. I recommend it especially to pregnant women because it relaxes them and the baby in the womb. Riding bicycles is also a great cardiovascular sport and I highly recommend to go to parks or less crowded streets because breathing in vehicle fumes can counteract the purpose of the bicycle riding benefits.

Some people like to run long distances. I personally do not believe running is as beneficial as walking at a quick pace because it may wear down our knees. Walking is one of the best things to do to stay healthy and live to a good, ripe age.

Now, another beautiful way to keep our bodies, bones, muscles and spirits flowing is by dancing. If you can join a dancing school and learn waltz, samba, merengue, salsa, tango, flamenco, and even belly dancing, they are all very beneficial for us and loads of fun. In these dancing styles, our passions may flow and we will feel totally in tune with our Universe.

Chapter Five
MEDITATE

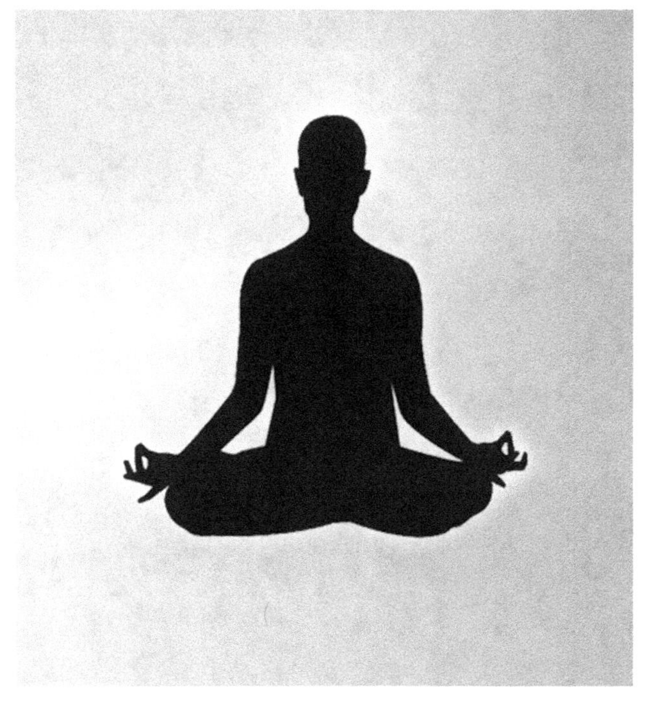

Meditation is a very important part of our busy lives because it is a time when we can return to our center, a time for our inner observance and peace.

A good time to meditate is upon awakening in the morning or after coming home from work at night. Some people find it easy to sit for about 20 minutes on the floor or on their beds on a pillow with their legs crossed and think of nothing but their breath. Others find it extremely hard to stand still and just breathe. A good alternative is to do walking meditation. That means, to walk, enjoy your environment: the sky, the trees, plants and occasional little animals that we see like birds, dogs, cats and squirrels. Just breathe in and out evenly and leave all your work and worries of the day behind you. If you walk in the evening and it's dark, enjoy looking at the stars and breathe in the oxygen from the trees. You will feel very renewed and will be ready for a restful sleep ahead.

It will be beneficial to have your dinner first and then go for a walk so that your food may digest nicely on your way.

The best thing to do is to leave your cell phone at home because nowadays, we are bombarded with electronics, media and information. Just enjoy nature and simply "be" instead of "do".

One of the secrets to longevity is to be outdoors and to do outdoor activities as much as possible because the fresh air renews our cells and keeps us happy.

Another way to meditate is to pray. At home or while walking, we can pray to the higher power of our belief and be thankful for everyone and everything we have in our lives. If we have a roof over our head, a family, a job, food and water at home, own a car, bike or bicycle and some electronic gadgets, we can surely consider ourselves millionaires in comparison to other people living in this world who have almost nothing. So we should be ever grateful for such gifts.

We can pray for others and their well being, which is a lovely way to meditate, not only because we are asking for their healing but also because we are remembering them in our prayers. With our busy lifestyles, we tend to forget to think of others and focus on our chores and ourselves. Let's think of our parents, grandparents, siblings, children, grandchildren, friends and all our brothers and sisters sharing this beautiful planet.

Some people meditate while washing dishes, with the flow of the running tap water or while doing laundry and folding the dry clothes (that's me by the way).
Still others meditate while cleaning the house or watering the garden, if they have one.

Lying on your bed and listening to soft, soothing music is yet another form of lovely meditation.

Whatever method works for you, choose one or a few and do it. You will feel energized and peaceful afterwards.

Chapter Six
REST

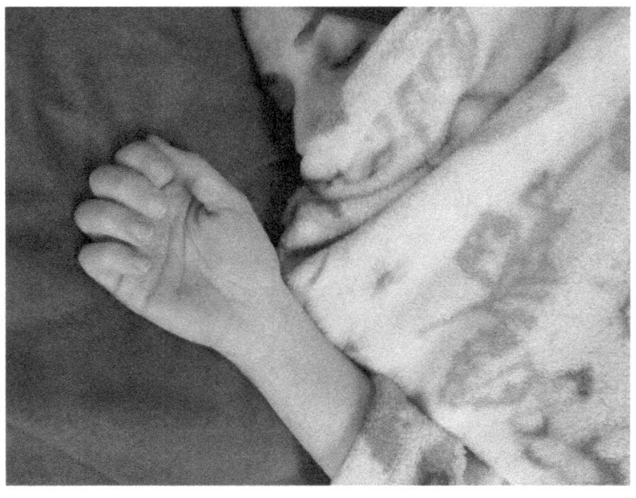

If you follow all of my advice in this book up to this point every day, you should be able to get a restful sleep.

One thing that you must have though, is a good mattress and a good pillow, something comfortable for you. Some people need very soft beds, others somewhat firm and others very firm, so always try your mattresses before purchasing them. Your sheets and pillow covers should preferably be made of cotton.

You should not sleep close to cell phones or TV's as they have electromagnetic fields and may interfere with our sleep patterns and therefore, we cannot sleep well.

Also, try to go to bed before 11 pm if you can and then wake up at around 6 or 7 am. Your body will adjust to these hours and you may even not need an alarm to wake you up because your inner clock will wake you. If you go to sleep after midnight, your sleeping hormone melatonin may not work well so you will probably not be able to rest properly and will wake up feeling tired.

Remember to stop eating at least two hours before bed time because people who eat and go straight to bed, start suffering from obesity, type II diabetes and heart disease. The reason is because your body cannot digest the food well, so

it lingers in the body, converts to sugar and settles in places not needed such as the belly.
Do not snack on sugary foods either because they are not only unhealthy for you, but they will give you a sudden boost of energy and you will not be able to rest.

Brush and floss your teeth, wash your face with a warm cloth, comb your hair and put on a nice and comfortable, loose pajama, preferably made of 100% cotton so that your pores may breathe easily.

Think of good thoughts, give thanks for your day, remember all the positive things that have happened, breathe out anything bad or upsetting, close your eyes and sleep.
Zzzzzzz!

Chapter Seven
SMILE

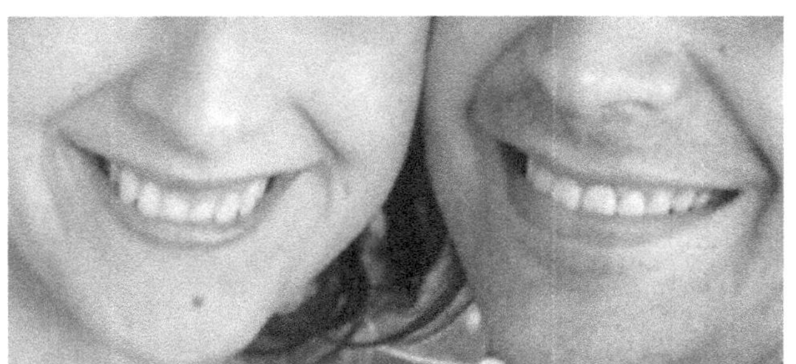

Now, you wake up in the morning refreshed and joyful because you have breathed deeply, drunk healthy drinks, your food was very nourishing, you exercised, meditated and rested.

You smile and keep on smiling as you do your morning chores.

Visualize all your internal organs smiling too, that is, your liver, gall bladder, heart, lungs, kidneys, stomach, intestines, pancreas and spleen. When you do this practice, any organ that may be in pain, may gradually start to feel better and if you feel good, you will keep on feeling good.

When you leave your home, keep on smiling at the world around you, the people you encounter and at yourself. Smiling has healing and calming benefits and even when you are not in the mood, just smiling can soothe you inside and out.

Smiles bring people together. Imagine the whole world smiling at the same time. What a magical healing moment for everyone that would be!

CONCLUSION

Breathe, drink, eat, exercise, meditate, rest and smile.

When we take care of our bodies and minds, then our spirits rejoice.

When we feel well, we feel enthusiastic about everything we do which leads us to care more for ourselves, for others and for our beautiful blue planet and all its life forms.

The ripple effect of our caring spreads around the world and then the Earth becomes a place of love, peace, forgiveness and understanding. Our collective consciousness is raised to a higher frequency where our lives become a living prayer and we and our planet are healed.